Praise for

LADYBUG YOGA

"We are delighted to have Ladybug Yoga as a part of our enrichment program. It is a fantastic program and our kids enjoy it immensely. The teachers are dynamic and they understand the needs of the children perfectly. The Ladybug Yoga classes are fun, creative, and our children are happy to participate!

"There is a reason that this program is termed 'enrichment.' Ladybug Yoga enriches the lives of all the children who participate in it. It is an extremely positive program and the children learn how to connect with themselves in a friendly, relaxed environment. This is learning, at its optimum.

"I would highly recommend Ladybug Yoga Classes!"

—Mike Jacobs, Saint Andrew's School

"Ladybug Yoga has now been in our school for over six years. Children at our school thrive and look forward to each and every class. This program is very creative, lots of fun, and, more important, it teaches children simple tools to use at home and in school which help them with self-confidence and concentration, among many other positive benefits. I highly recommend Ladybug Yoga to schools and to parents. The results are astounding!"

—Nancy Goldstein, Early Childhood Center Director,
B'nai Torah Congregation

"For the past year, my three-year-old daughter has been taking Ladybug Yoga classes as a weekly after-school enrichment activity. She looks forward to 'yoga day' each week, and she is all smiles when she comes home. She enjoys demonstrating the various yoga positions she learns each week (downward-facing dog, tree pose, etc.), and telling us about the latest lessons with her friends in class.

"Over the past year, my daughter's balance and agility have improved dramatically. I attribute it in no small part to the Ladybug Yoga classes, which have given her age-appropriate methods to focus on her body and coordination. I appreciate that Ladybug Yoga also teaches her mindfulness and relaxation techniques, which carry over from class into her everyday routine.

"Ladybug Yoga provides a safe, fun, and enriching experience for my daughter, and the lessons will grow with her as she matures. I look forward to having her continue Ladybug Yoga classes in the future."

—Nicole K., South Florida

"I'm so grateful to Ladybug Yoga. After my daughter started taking classes, she really learned how to calm herself with the breathing techniques she learned. Whether it was to calm herself during a tantrum or when she felt anxious, she now does her breathing techniques or takes herself on a 'relaxation journey' as she does in class. It is so inspiring to see. I myself do yoga and wish I could've started at her young age. Such useful tools to deal with lifelong situations! Not only that, but her balance has increased, as well as her flexibility. She also dances and plays tennis, and I can't say enough good things about how these yoga classes have helped to improve her body condition and excel in her other activities. My daughter is much happier, which makes me one happy mommy! Thanks again, Ladybug Yoga!"

—Stacy J., South Florida

LADYBUG
YOGA

AT-HOME PARENTS
TOOLS & TECHNIQUES GUIDE

SANDY GOLOGURSKY

Founder, Ladybug Yoga LLC

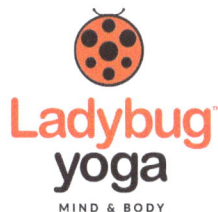

Ladybug
yoga
MIND & BODY

DISCLAIMER: The information provided in this book is intended for parents and teachers to use at home or in the classroom for short intervals throughout the day. All forms of physical activity and exercise carry with them a risk of injury, and not all yoga practices and poses are suitable for everyone. Parents and teachers must use their judgment and discretion during each session, with safety being paramount.

The author, Ladybug Yoga LLC, and its affiliates assume no responsibility or liability for any injuries or losses that might result from practicing yoga or engaging in any of the activities contained within this book. Should the reader have any questions concerning the appropriateness of any exercise or activity described, the author and Ladybug Yoga strongly suggest consulting a certified yoga instructor.

Published by
Ladybug Yoga LLC
Boca Raton, FL
www.theLadybugYoga.com
E-mail: Sandy@theladybugyoga.com
Facebook/LadybugYoga
Instagram/LadybugYoga

ISBN: 978-0-69298-244-0

Production by The Book Couple • www.thebookcouple.com

Contents

About Ladybug Yoga 2

Incorporating Ladybug Yoga into Your Home 3

Ladybug Yoga Body Awareness Time 6

Ladybug Yoga Breathing Exercises 7

Ladybug Yoga Poses 10

Ladybug Yoga Games 17

Take a Ladybug Yoga Moment 20

Ladybug Yoga Positive Affirmations 22

Ladybug Yoga Guided Relaxations 23

A Note from Sandy, *Founder of Ladybug Yoga* 25

About the Author 27

Continue the Learning 28

About Ladybug Yoga

LADYBUG YOGA is a unique children's yoga program that has been taught in yoga studios, preschools, private schools, charter schools, private classes, and summer camps throughout South Florida since 2009. We have witnessed that teaching these amazing tools to young children will build a positive foundation for their whole life. This program is designed for children ages 3 and up and utilizes practical tools that have no basis in any particular religious faith.

Yoga helps children develop important skills in a fun, non-competitive environment. Even at a young age, children often feel pressure at school academically and socially, plus the added stress of competitive organized sports makes it easy for boys and girls to become overly self-critical and lose confidence in themselves as they grow and change.

Our goal is to nurture a child's inner strength and self-acceptance while encouraging and challenging them to develop the following attributes:

- Strength
- Coordination
- Flexibility
- Concentration
- Sense of Calm

- Balance
- Body Awareness
- Better Focus
- Self-confidence

Incorporating Ladybug Yoga into Your Home

With our children's schedules being so overwhelming these days—filled with homework and after-school programs—plus all their regular responsibilities, doesn't give them much time to stop and have a full yoga class during each day . . . but that's okay! Practicing yoga for even a few minutes each day is highly beneficial for children.

When incorporating the Ladybug Yoga tools and techniques into your home, allow your child(den) to be creative with their body movements. Encourage your children to "shine as bright" as they can!

Explain to your child(ren) the importance of these tools and techniques. Once they are familiar, ask them every day, "Why is it important to do yoga?"

Here are some responses to discuss with your child(ren):

◆ Stay healthy

◆ Be happy

◆ Get strong muscles

◆ Learn to calm our minds and bodies

◆ Stretch our bodies to become more flexible while we grow

◆ Learn how to balance

◆ Help focus at school and while doing homework (concentration)

◆ Learn how to be aware of how our body is feeling (body awareness)

◆ Feel good and proud of ourselves (self-esteem)

Suggestions for when to incorporate Ladybug Yoga into your home:

- First thing in the morning
- After school
- Before bed
- Long car ride/ airplane ride
- For a family activity
- As an exercise
- When you need a break
- When not listening to parents
- When feeling stressed
- When feeling overwhelmed
- When feeling anxious
- When feeling sad
- When feeling angry
- When feeling tired
- When feeling unmotivated
- When lacking focus or concentration
- When unable to fall asleep
- When not listening to parents
- During a tantrum
- During an argument between siblings
- Just for fun

AT-HOME YOGA SET-UP

Depending on the available time and circumstances, you can implement any or all of the following suggestions:

- Choose a setting that will limit distractions.
- Turn off lights, allowing only natural light to come in.
- Play Ladybug Yoga class music to create a relaxing atmosphere.
- Sit crisscross on your yoga mat or on any comfortable surface.

LADYBUG YOGA ESSENTIALS

The following items are recommended for the practice of yoga in the home. All items are available through www.theLadybugYoga.com.

◆ Ladybug Yoga Mat

◆ Ladybug Yoga Class Music (USB, mp3 format)

◆ Ladybug Yoga Recorded Guided Crystal Journey
(USB, mp3 format)

◆ Ladybug Yoga Crystals

◆ Ladybug Yoga What's-in-the-Box? Game

◆ Ladybug Yoga Ladybugs Game

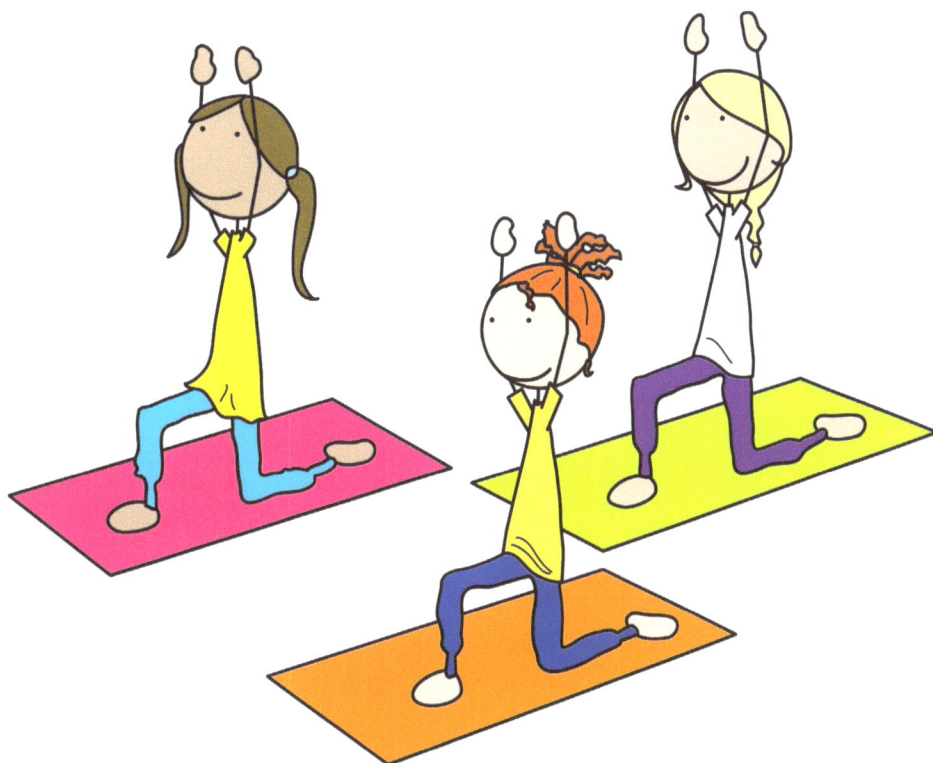

Ladybug Yoga Body Awareness Time

BODY AWARENESS

Here is an amazing opportunity for your child(ren) and it will only take about 30 seconds. As children become more aware of their bodies, it quickly calms them down and brings them into the present moment. This awareness enables them to relax, so they can move on with their day more calmly and with more focus.

Have your child(ren) sit crisscross on their yoga mat or on any comfortable surface with hands on knees. Parent says "Close your eyes. I want you to wiggle your toes (pause). Wiggle your fingers (pause). Wiggle your nose (pause). Put a beautiful smile on your face (pause). Feel your breath in your body (pause). Take a big inhale through your nose, making a big balloon in your belly, then exhale through your nose, letting it go. (Repeat breath 2 more times.) Now slowly open your eyes."

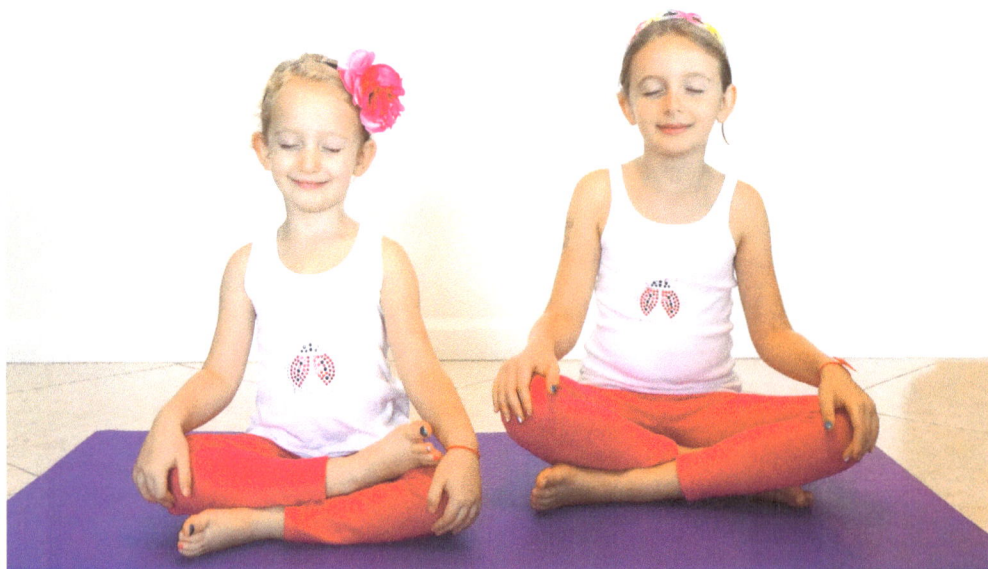

Ladybug Yoga Breathing Exercises

Breathing practice is very important for many reasons. To name a few: Breathing teaches children to turn inwardly and connect within themselves to experience, feel, gain control of, and understand their bodies. Breathing practice also trains their bodies to respond automatically to help calm themselves down at times when they are feeling stressed, anxious, or sad. Focused and correct forms of breathing are related to many positive benefits, including health, vitality, and happiness. By learning this important tool at a young age, children will have received the best gift possible for life!

Choose one breathing exercise per session.
Time frame: 30 seconds to 5 minutes

Breathing exercises are done through the nose only, unless guided otherwise. Inhale through the nose, then exhale through the nose.

Inhale: Take a deep breath in through your nose.

Exhale: Release the breath out through your nose.

Hold: Hold the breath for the count.

BALLOON BREATH

◆ Have your child(ren) lie on their back on their yoga mat with hands on their belly. As children inhale, they push their belly into their hands, making a BIG balloon. As they exhale, they let the balloon deflate. (Repeat for 4–5 breaths.)

◆ Then, inhale and hold their balloon in their belly for a count of 3, then exhale, letting that breath out. Increase the length of the breath hold each time to make the exercise more challenging. (Repeat 5 times)

◆ Some children may do the reverse with their breath and belly, so assist by placing your hands over theirs and encourage them to push their belly into your hands as they inhale.

SIGH BREATH

◆ Have your child(ren) sit crisscross on their yoga mat with hands on knees.

◆ Parent says, "Big inhale through your nose and exhale out through your mouth, making a loud sighing noise." (Repeat 4–8 times.)

◆ Parent explains that when we breathe in, we breathe in happiness and other good feelings, and that when we breathe out, we can let out any anger, sadness, or stress we may be feeling.

◆ Have your child(ren) suggest something to inhale and something to exhale.

STRETCH BREATH

◆ Have your child(ren) lie on their back on their yoga mat with legs outstretched and arms by their sides.

◆ Parent says, "Inhale through your nose as we stretch our arms overhead and stretch our toes away from our body, getting a nice stretch. Exhale out of your mouth, arms come back down by your side." (Repeat 3 times.)

◆ Parent says, "Stretch your left arm and left leg, then your right arm and right leg."

◆ Add a hold as both arms are stretched overhead. Increase the length of the breath hold each time to make the exercise more challenging. (Repeat 5 times.)

WAVE BREATH

◆ Have your child(ren) sit crisscross on their yoga mat.

◆ Demonstrating with hand movements, parent asks, "Does a wave go up and down or side to side?"

◆ Child(ren) will answer "up and down." Parent says, "Great, so let's make waves with our hands a few times. Place your hands in front of you and draw them up, up, up and down, down, down." (Repeat 2 times.) "Now let's add the breath with our hands moving. Inhale, the wave goes up—overhead—and exhale, the wave comes down." (Repeat 4 times.) "Add a hold as the wave is up in the sky." Increase holds each time. (Repeat 3–5 times.)

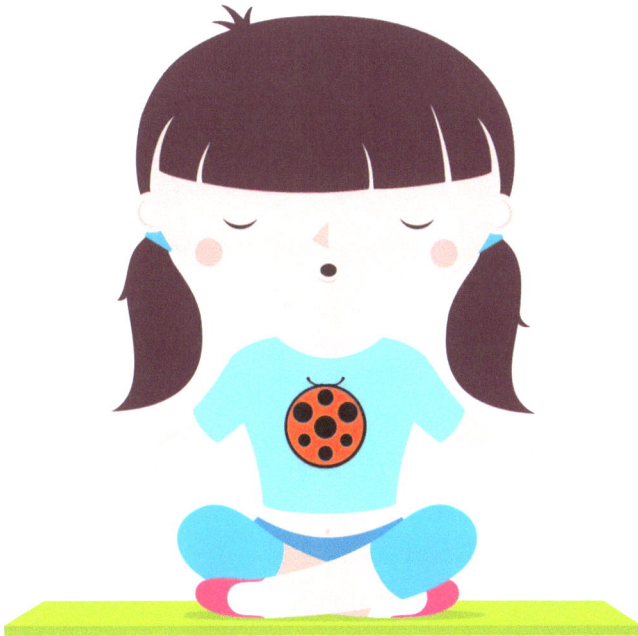

Ladybug Yoga Poses

The practice of yoga poses is very important, as the poses have many beneficial effects. Children develop strength, flexibility, and balance, while discovering that their minds and bodies are connected, which assists them in increasing their self-awareness, building their self-esteem, and helping them learn how to focus and concentrate.

The **Ladybug Yoga Poses** are designed for children of different ages. Each child has a different range of flexibility. It is important that the parent is always conscious of each child's limitations and supports them at all levels while practicing the poses.

The symbol(s) next to each pose indicate its suggested age-appropriate level(s): **P** Preschool, **E+** Elementary and up.

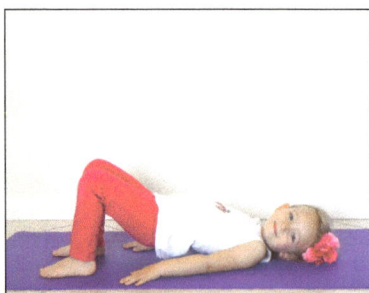

Bridge Pose (P, E+)—Bend legs and place feet flat on floor; lift hips up and bring them back down. (Older children can hold ankles or heels for a count of 10–20.)

Parent says, "Let the boats come through" or "Let a big cruise ship come through, so lift really high" or "Let a small canoe come through, so just lift a little."

Candle Pose (Shoulder Stand) (P, E+)—Stretch legs up to the sky and twinkle (wiggle) toes. (Older children can lift into shoulder stand, supporting lower back, while twinkling their toes.)

Parent and child(ren) sing, "Twinkle, Twinkle, Little Star."

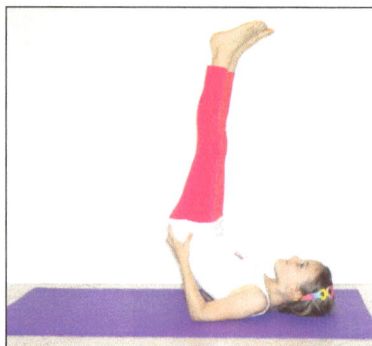

Tiny Ball Pose (P, E+)—Hug knees into a tiny ball, and rock from side to side.

Parent asks, "Who can get into the smallest ball?"

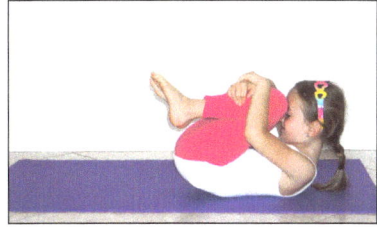

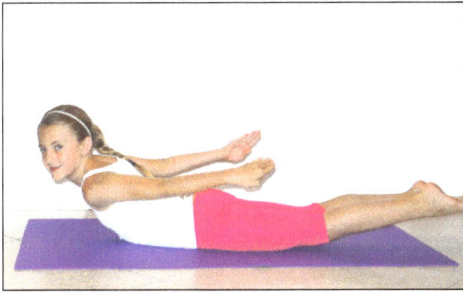

Superman Pose (P, E+)—Lie on stomach, extend arms out in front on mat. At the same time, lift arms, legs, and head off mat. With straight arms, sweep arms behind until fingers are pointing away from body. Fly like Superman!

Butterfly Pose (P, E+)—Place soles of feet together, flapping knees, with hands on shoulders or on head as antennas. (Older children place hands on feet.)

Parent asks, "Where are we traveling?" or "What color is your butterfly today?"

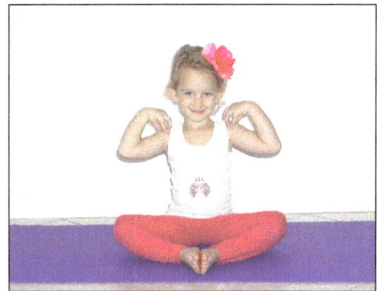

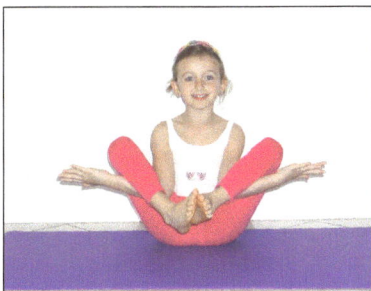

Flower Pose (P, E+)—Begin in Butterfly Pose. With knees up, place arms through legs and support knees. Lift legs off floor, keeping toes together, and find balance.

Parent asks, "What type of flower are you today?" or "What color flower are you?" or says, "Let's hold and count to 10."

Twist Pose (P, E+)—Extend legs forward. Bend right leg and plant foot on floor close to body and give knee a big hug with left arm. Stretch right arm up to the sky, wave hello, and then place it behind back close to body. Twist to look over right shoulder to see what is behind you. Repeat on the other side.

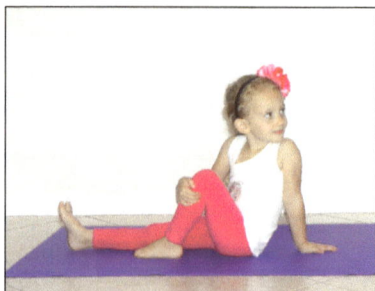

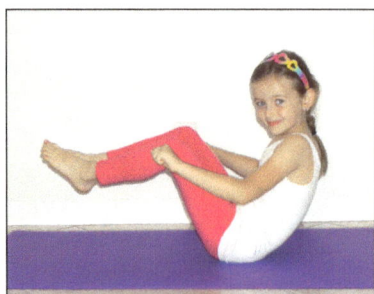

Boat Pose (P, E+)—Legs together, bend legs and bring feet off the floor, placing knees and feet parallel to the floor. Arms at the sides, moving as if rowing a boat. (Older children hold for a count of 10–20.)

Parent and children sing "Row Your Boat."

Baby Pose (P, E+)—Begin on knees with tops of feet flat on floor, then sit backside on heels, and bring head to the ground with arms along sides.

Parent asks, "What do babies say?" Wah!

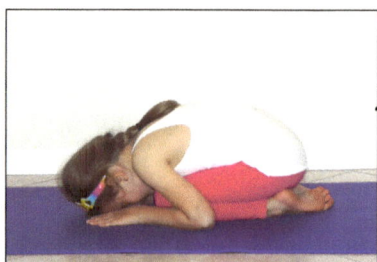

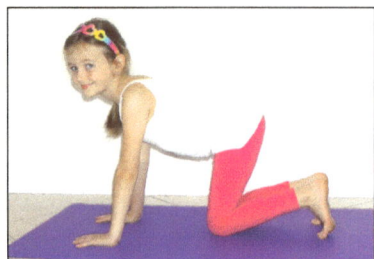

Cow Pose (P, E+)—Begin on hands and knees, then drop hips and shoulders back and look forward with chin slightly raised.

Parent asks, "What do cows say?" Mooooo!

Cat Pose (P, E+)—Begin on hands and knees, then round back, bringing chin to chest.

Parent asks, "What do cats say?" Meowwwww!

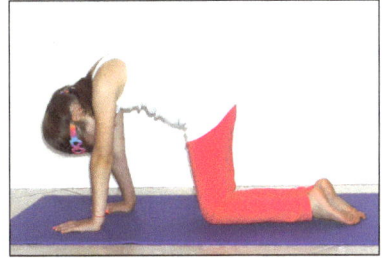

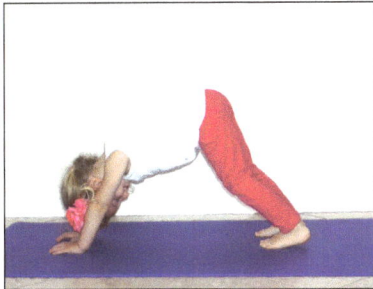

Dog Pose (P, E+)—Place hands under shoulders on the mat and lift hips to the sky with heels on the floor, eyes looking at knees. (Older children can lift one leg up, and then switch with the other leg. Then lift one leg and opposite hand, then switch.)

Parent asks, "What does a dog say?" Woof! Woof!

Snake Pose (P, E+)—Begin on hands and knees, and bring hips forward onto the floor and lift chest, shoulders, and back.

Parent asks, "What do snakes say?" Sssssssssss!

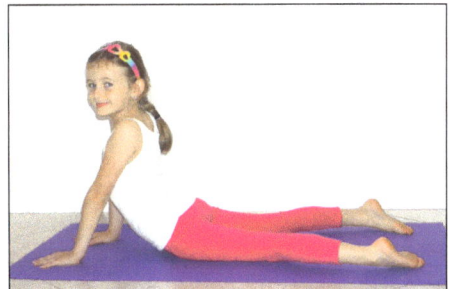

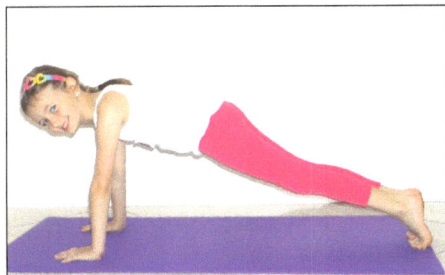

Plank Pose (P, E+)—Begin on hands and knees, and curl toes under, lift knees off the floor, walking feet back to create a straight plank. Hold for a count of 10–30.

Parent asks, "Who can be as straight as can be?"

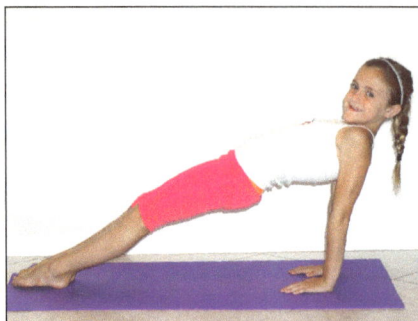

Slide Pose (Reverse Plank) (P, E+)—
Sit on mat with legs together, extended out front. Place hands behind body with fingers facing body and shoulder blades and elbows drawn together. Lift bottom off the floor, straightening arms and lifting chest. Point toes to the floor. Hold for a count of 10.

"Wheeee! Down the slide we go!"

Mountain Pose (P, E+)—Stand with legs together and arms by sides and hold to be a tall mountain. Then take one hand and shield eyes, as if looking down at something.

Parent says, "Stay very still and tall like a mountain."

Parent asks, "What's at the bottom of your mountain?"

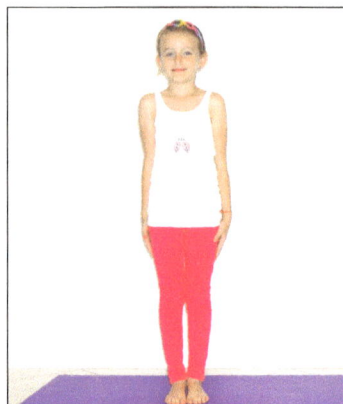

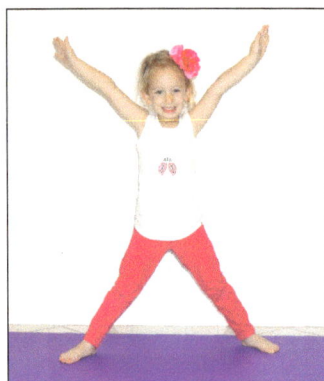

Shining Star Pose (P, E+)—Standing in Mountain Pose, jump arms and legs open to a shining star and smile. Hold. Then jump arms and legs together, back to Mountain Pose. Do this several times like jumping jacks.

Parent says, "Smile like a shining star and hold."
Parent says, "Open and close, open and close."
(Repeating and progressing faster each time.)

Forward Fold Touching Toes Pose (P, E+)—
Standing in Mountain Pose, extend arms to the sky. Fold forward, touching toes, and hold for a count of 10. Roll all the way up.

Parent says, "I'm touching my toes. Are you touching yours?"

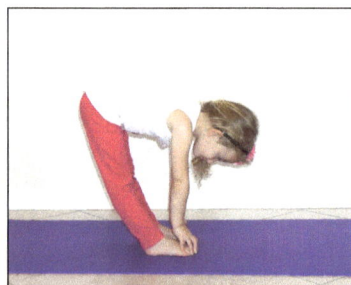

Chair Pose (P, E+)—Stand with feet hip-width apart and bend knees, dropping hips back and pretending to be sitting on a chair. Extend arms out front by ears.

Parent asks, "Who's sitting in your chair?"

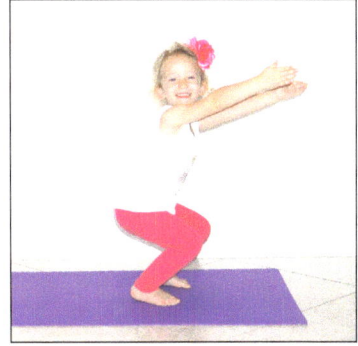

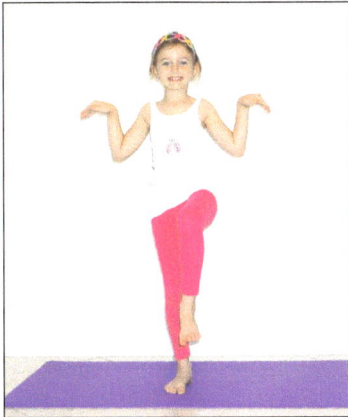

Flamingo Pose (P, E+)—Standing in Mountain Pose, lift knee up, bringing thigh parallel to floor. Bend arms, placing elbows to body and hands facing out as wings. Balance on one side, then hop and switch to the other leg. Balance on that side, then switch. (Older children lift knee and hold as high as they can for a count of 10–20.)

Parent says, "Hop, hop, hop." Parent asks, "What color is a flamingo?"

Tree Pose (P, E+)—Lift one foot up and place on thigh and place palms together to heart center. When balanced, extend arms up to create branches on a tree. Repeat on the other side and wave branches from side to side.

Parent says, "Pick a spot to stare at and find your balance." Or "It's a windy day and our branches are swaying."

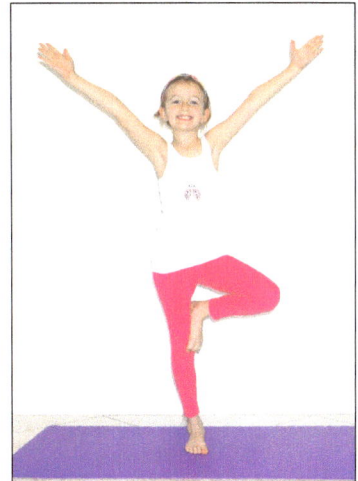

Elephant Pose (Warrior 2) (P, E+)—Open legs into a V and extend one knee over ankle and open arms parallel to floor using front arm as trunk, placed in front of chin, and back arm as tail, swaying trunk. Repeat on the other side. (Older children hold pose with straight arms parallel to the floor for a count of 20.)

Parent says, "Heee, heee!"

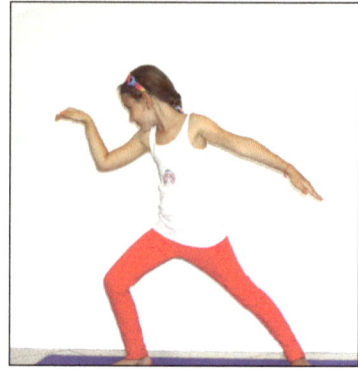

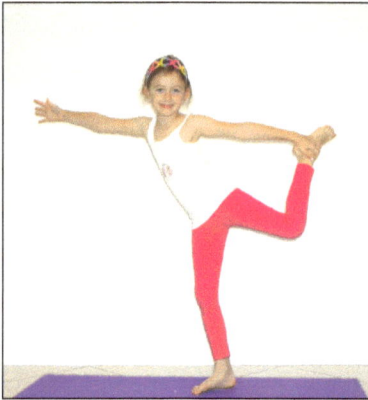

Dancer Pose (P, E+)—Standing in Mountain Pose, bend and lift one leg behind body, grabbing the foot. Extend opposite arm in front of body, reaching up to the sky, slightly leaning forward, and arching back while pushing foot into hand. Repeat on the other side.

Parent says, "Dancer! Dancer!"

Triangle Pose (P, E+)—Open legs into a V shape and drop one arm, holding onto thigh, knee, or shin, extending other arm up to the sky while looking up. Repeat on the other side.

Parent says, "Triangle."

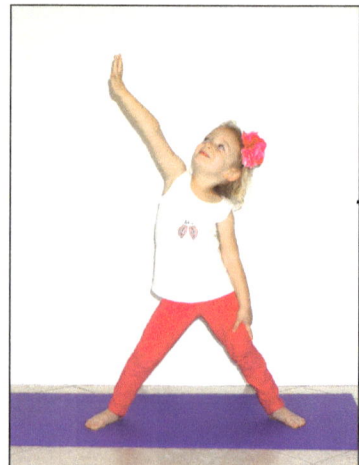

Ladybug Yoga Games

Each **Ladybug Yoga Game** incorporates various yoga poses found in this manual. Games are a time to have fun and interact with one another while receiving all the beneficial effects of the yoga poses. When deciding together which games to play during your session, it is best to offer a variety of games. Play as time permits. Games with an asterisk (*) indicate Ladybug Yoga Essentials, available from www.theLadybugYoga.com.

BRIDGE GAME ⓟ ⓔ Ⓜ

Create a long bridge by lining up mini yoga mats on the floor. Parent says, "We are going to the jungle today, and we will be different animals crossing the bridge. But don't fall into the water!" Have your child(ren) cross the bridge, imitating an animal pose. Once they have crossed the bridge, they walk around the mats to the beginning. (Do this 4–6 times for different animals.) Next, have your child(ren) make up whatever animal pose they want to imitate while crossing the bridge. (Do this 4–6 times.)

CREATE SEQUENCE GAME (P, E+)

Parent creates and demonstrates a sequence with 4–8 yoga poses. Have your child(ren) do the sequence, trying to remember them and perform them in order. Then have your child(ren) take a turn creating a sequence.

DO THAT POSE GAME (P, E+)

Parent names a yoga pose without demonstrating and child(ren) get into that pose. Parent continues with different yoga poses until the child(ren) cannot demonstrate one. Then reverse roles and let your child(ren) name the poses.

HOLDING YOGA POSE GAME (P, E+)

Parent chooses an appropriately challenging yoga pose. Have your child(ren) get into that pose and hold it for as long as they can. If your child(ren) have been holding the pose for a while, count to 10 have them come out of the pose. Repeat with different yoga poses.

KANGAROO HOPPING GAME* (P, E+)

Set up Ladybug Yoga Mini Yoga Mats close together, like a bridge, but not touching. Have your child(ren) hop like a kangaroo from mat to mat. At the end, have them walk around the mats back to start. For the next round, parent moves the mats further apart to make the game more challenging. (Do this several times, making it more challenging each time.)

LADYBUG YOGA LADYBUGS GAME* (P, E+)

Hide the ladybugs around the room while your child(ren) aren't looking. When all the ladybugs have been hidden, have your child(ren) walk around the room in various traveling animal poses. Parent tells a story to lead the animals around the jungle, and then, when they get very hungry for dinner, they need to search for the ladybugs as their food. Parent says, "Time for dinner!" and the child(ren) start searching for the hidden ladybugs and pretending to eat them. Repeat with different traveling animals.

LADYBUG YOGA WHAT'S IN THE BOX? GAME* (P, E+)

Parent shows the children the special Ladybug Yoga box and says, "What's in the box? What's in the box?" Parent places the box near the child(ren) on the floor. Take turns picking a card from the box without looking. Follows the request on the card.

YES I CAN GAME (P, E+)

Have your child(ren) with legs together and open arms overhead, forming a Y with their body, representing the word "YES." Have your child(ren) say a positive affirmation beginning with "Yes, I can . . ." out loud, with energy and pride. For example: "Yes, I can dive into a swimming pool!" or "Yes, I can tie my shoes!" or "Yes, I can ride a bicycle!"

YOGA POSE MEMORY GAME (P)

Parent demonstrates a yoga pose, and the child(ren) does that yoga pose and adds another pose. Play continues, adding more and more poses, until child(ren) and parent feel challenged to remember.

YOGI SAYS (P, E+)

This is a variation of the game Simon Says. Instead of the command "Simon says," parent uses the command "Yogi says." Have your child(ren) stand on their yoga mat facing you. Parent says and demonstrates (for example) "Yogi says tree," or "Yogi says baby," and so on. Child(ren) get into the pose that "Yogi says."

If parent says, "dog," but doesn't say, "Yogi says dog," child(ren) are not supposed to go into that pose. Parent says, "Listen carefully and only do poses when Yogi says." Play continues until your child(ren) can perform sequences correctly. If there is time, your child(ren) can take turns being Yogi.

YOGI STATUE AND ARTIST GAME (P, E+)

Note: Pencils (or crayons) and drawing paper are needed for this activity. Work as partners. One partner is the yogi statue (holds a yoga pose), and one partner is the artist (draws the yogi statue). After enough time has passed for artists to draw their statues, switch roles.

Take a Ladybug Yoga Moment

Below are **Ladybug Yoga Moments**. If you have 5–10 minutes and want to combine breathing with yoga poses, here are your go-to "moments." Pick one Moment to follow and repeat the steps as time permits. Combination poses are for children to switch back and forth to create a flow of energy in their bodies.

At the end of the chosen Moment, have your child(ren) pick a Ladybug Yoga Positive Affirmation to recite aloud (page 22). After completing the Affirmation, finish with Ladybug Yoga Body Awareness Time (page 6).

#1 Moment

◆ 3 Balloon Breaths.

◆ 3 Dog & Snake combination poses.

◆ Chair Pose. Hold for a count of 10.

◆ Flamingo Pose. Find balance on each side.

#2 Moment

◆ 3 Stretch Breaths.

◆ 3 Tiny Ball & Butterfly combination poses.

◆ Plank Pose. Hold for a count of 10.

◆ Tree Pose. Find balance on each side.

#3 Moment

◆ 3 Sigh Breaths.

◆ 3 Baby & Bridge combination poses.

◆ Flower Pose. Hold for a count of 10.

◆ Dancer Pose. Find balance on each side.

#4 Moment

◆ 3 Wave Breaths.

◆ 3 Cat & Cow combination poses.

◆ Slide Pose. Hold for a count of 10.

◆ Flamingo Pose. Find balance on each side.

#5 Moment

- 3 Stretch Breaths.

- 3 Mountain & Forward Fold Touching Toes combination poses.

- Boat Pose. Hold for a count of 10.

- Tree Pose. Find balance on each side.

#6 Moment

- 3 Sigh Breaths.

- 3 Snake & Superman combination poses.

- Chair Pose. Hold for a count of 10.

- Flamingo Pose. Find balance on each side.

#7 Moment

- 3 Wave Breaths.

- 3 Shining Star & Triangle combination poses.

- Plank Pose. Hold for a count of 10.

- Dancer Pose. Find balance on each side.

#8 Moment

- 3 Balloon Breaths.

- 3 Elephant & Dog combination poses.

- Flower Pose. Hold for a count of 10.

- Tree Pose. Find balance on each side.

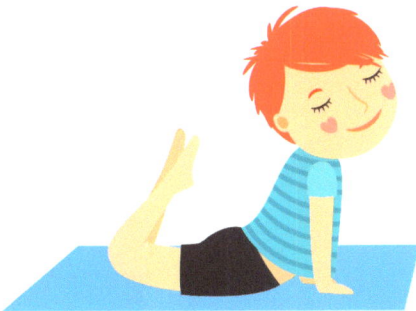
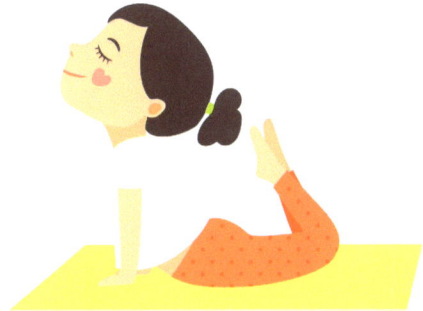

Ladybug Yoga Positive Affirmations

Positive affirmations are very important in our daily lives. Our thoughts create our feelings, which then ripple into our reality. It is important for children to learn this skill in order to focus on the beauty and positivity around and within themselves, as life will always offer challenges. Teaching children this tool will strengthen self-esteem and further the practice of mind over matter, which will assist them in overcoming obstacles they may encounter throughout their lives.

Parent chooses one Ladybug Yoga Positive Affirmation for the week or has child(ren) choose an affirmation of their own. Share this affirmation aloud each day.

In the game section, you will find the "YES I Can . . . Game." This is a fun game that helps to build self-esteem.

Here are some affirmations to share with your child(ren). Parent can also have their child(ren) suggest their own affirmations.

- I Am Happy
- I Am Strong
- I Am Funny
- I Am Loved
- I Am Smart

- I Am Brave
- I Believe in Myself
- I Am Beautiful
- I Am Caring

- I Am Sharing
- I Am Peaceful
- I Trust in Myself
- I Can Do It!

Ladybug Yoga Guided Relaxations

Relaxation is an essential component of the yoga class. During this time, children can fully surrender their bodies, as they are able to slow down and be in the present moment. By taking this time, they are allowing their bodies to balance and rejuvenate while calming their minds. Teaching children these tools for how to stay in a place of calmness can benefit them greatly in their daily lives.

Have your child(ren) hold a crystal in their hand or place it on their body while lying on their back. It is recommended that children not place them in their mouths, eyes, nose, ears, or inside their clothing. Tell your child(ren) to handle crystals with care.

Choose one guided relaxation to incorporate into each session.

CRYSTAL BODY

Have your child(ren) choose a crystal and lie on their back on their yoga mat. Parent puts on Ladybug Yoga Class Music* and turns off or dims the lights. Parent asks child(ren) to close their eyes.

Pausing for a moment between statements, parent says, "We are going to calm your body. So relax your toes. Relax your feet. Relax your ankles. Relax your legs. Relax your knees. Relax your hips. Relax your back. Relax your stomach. Relax your shoulders. Relax your arms. Relax your elbows. Relax your hands. Relax your fingers. Relax your neck. Relax your throat. Relax your head. Relax your eyes. Relax your ears. Relax your cheeks. Relax your nose. Relax your chin. Relax your mouth. Relax your teeth. Relax your tongue. Relax your hair. Relax your spine. Relax your whole body. Be calm. Relax your mind. Listen to the music and stay calm. You are all doing a wonderful job! Put a beautiful smile on your face. Just relax. Just relax." (Parent is silent for a few moments, then repeats, "Just relax. Just relax." Again, parent is silent for a few moments.)

Parent then says, "Slowly, I want you to wiggle your toes, wiggle your fingers, open your eyes, and stay calm. Stretch your arms overhead and get a nice stretch." Have your child(ren) sit criss-cross and share how they felt during their relaxation.

CRYSTAL JOURNEY

Have your child(ren) choose a crystal and lie on their back on their yoga mat. Parent puts on Ladybug Yoga Class Music* and turns off or dims the lights. Parent asks child(ren) to close their eyes. As option to using music and reciting the Crystal Journey, parent can play the Ladybug Yoga Recorded Guided Crystal Journey*.

Parent says, "Close your eyes. You are now going to travel with your crystal to your favorite place in the whole entire world. When I count to three, you will take off into the sky and travel to your favorite place in the world. One, two, three. You are now traveling through the sky, through the clouds. The wind is brushing through your hair, and you are getting closer to your favorite place. When I count down from three to one, you will land at your favorite place in the world. Three, two, one. You have now landed at your favorite place in the world with your crystal. It's time for you to do whatever your favorite thing is to do in your imagination, in your mind—whether it is to go on rides, sing, dance, eat, play, swim, relax, cook, color, or read. Whatever your favorite thing to do is, that is what you are doing now with your crystal, just you and your crystal." (Parent repeats this last line softly several times to keep the child(ren) in their favorite place for a while.)

Parent then says, "Now it is time to travel back to your yoga mat. When I count to three, you will take off into the sky. One, two, three. You are now traveling with your crystal through the clouds. The wind is brushing through your hair. When I count from three to one, you will land back on your yoga mat. Three, two, one."

Parent then says, "Slowly, I want you to wiggle your toes, wiggle your fingers, open your eyes, and stay calm. Stretch your arms overhead and get a nice stretch." Have your child(ren) sit criss-cross and share how they felt during their journey.

---

*These Ladybug Yoga Essentials are available at www.theLadybugYoga.com

A Note from Sandy
Founder of Ladybug Yoga

The **Ladybug Yoga** curriculum was created as an extension of my heart and soul. When I look back over my life, I see two main themes developing: the first is my role as a natural yogi, and the second is my role as a compassionate teacher.

As a young child who was raised by a health-conscious mother, I was afforded the opportunity to sit in on many yoga classes. I remember enjoying the yoga classes, even at an early age, and feeling right at home in the yoga studio. Yoga became a passion for me early on.

My other passion was being a role model and caretaker for young kids. I spent many summers working as a camp counselor, and after graduating high school, I became an Early Childhood Educator and taught for a few years. I adored working with children in this realm, but felt that an important piece of teaching was missing for me. I knew deep inside that I needed to expand on my formal training as an ECE and learn more about the ancient practice of yoga that I had been exposed to.

In 2004, after leaving Canada and moving to Florida to join my family, I found a highly revered yoga teacher training program: Nosara Yoga Institute in Costa Rica. Upon completing my RYT-200 (Registered Yoga Teacher) certification, I returned home and completed my RCYT (Registered Children's Yoga Teacher) training. I began teaching both adults and children in local yoga studios. I was extremely fortunate to have had the support and ongoing teachings of an amazing mentor who took me under her wing and guided me to flourish.

In 2009—when my first daughter, Maya, was born—it all came together for me, and I was inspired to combine my Early Childhood Education with my yoga training. That was exactly the instant—the "aha!" moment—in which **Ladybug Yoga** was created! I set out to create an original children's yoga program that teaches the most incredible, practical tools that kids can use in their everyday lives.

Other teachers soon joined me for the **Ladybug Yoga** adventure. We have been teaching children three years and older in schools and facilities throughout South Florida. As a result, the children, their parents, and the schools have witnessed firsthand how kids can benefit from such a curriculum.

I've received an abundance of interest from yoga instructors, teachers, parents, schools, and therapists to learn our program so that they can implement its lessons and tools in their own work with children, as well as with their own children at home. This interest led to my second "aha!" moment: I realized that it was time to create this program, which I now have the pleasure of presenting to you. This labor of love has evolved over the years into the Ladybug Yoga curriculum, and I invite you to share it with the children in your life.

—Sandy Gologursky, ECE, E-RYT 200, RCYT, YACEP

About the Author

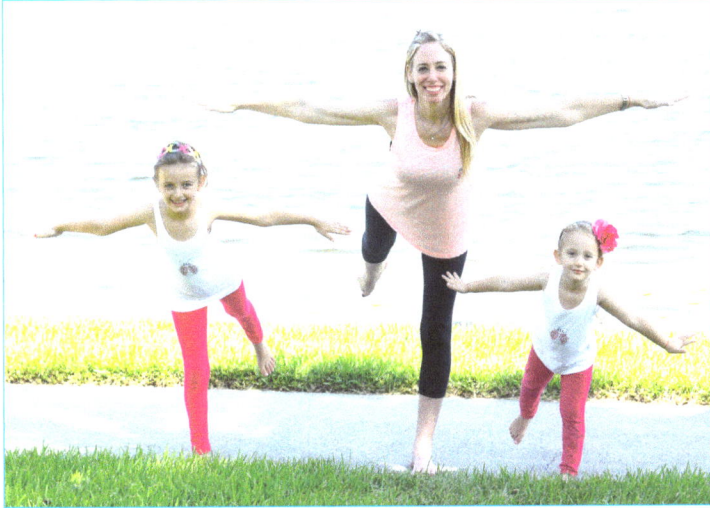

Sandy Gologursky, ECE, E-RYT 200, RCYT, YACEP, is the creator of the Ladybug Yoga system. She is a passionate advocate for Yoga practice for children. She believes that providing appropriate tools to parents and teachers will help them to make a positive difference in the lives of children as they grow and develop.

Contact Sandy at contact@LadybugYoga.com
or visit www.theLadybugYoga.com

Continue the Learning

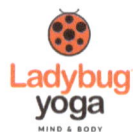

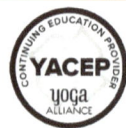

Ladybug Yoga is here to provide you with various guides and workshops for you to continue learning, which will truly assist you in your journey of sharing these amazing tools and techniques with children. Here are our recommended workshops & guides to further your education, all available at www.theLadybugYoga.com:

LADYBUG YOGA CHILDREN'S TEACHER TRAINING (IN-PERSON / ONLINE)*

Ladybug Yoga Children's Teacher Training is a dynamic, interactive, and fun training program geared toward anyone seeking to work with or currently working with children.

Expand your business, grow your clientele, and add a new branch of teaching by learning our practical, useful tools and techniques that will enable you to share the benefits of yoga with children to help them in their everyday lives!

After completion of this training, you will feel confident and excited to share these incredible new skills with children!

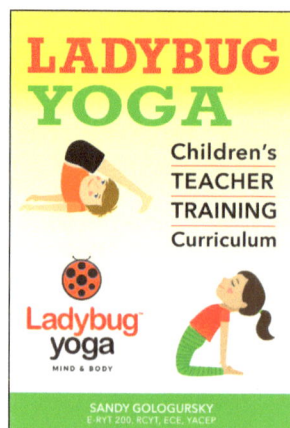

LADYBUG YOGA IN-CLASSROOM TEACHER TOOLS & TECHNIQUES GUIDE

Ladybug Yoga In-Classroom Teacher Tools & Techniques is a creative and useful go-to guide that assists school teachers in implementing these useful tools and techniques with their children.

We understand that classroom schedules are so full of daily activities that it would be challenging to add a full yoga class into the school day . . . but thats okay! Practicing yoga for even a few minutes each day is highly beneficial for both children and teachers.

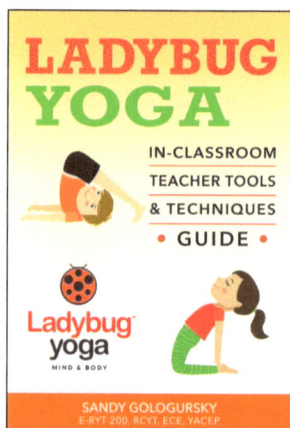

LADYBUG YOGA 8-WEEK SESSION PROGRAM PLAN

After completing the Ladybug Yoga Children's Teacher Training, it is now time for you to go out and positively impact the lives of children throughout the world!

Since it can be overwhelming or stressful at first to create your lesson plans, Ladybug Yoga created the **Ladybug Yoga 8-Week Session Program Plan** to make it easier on you from start to finish!

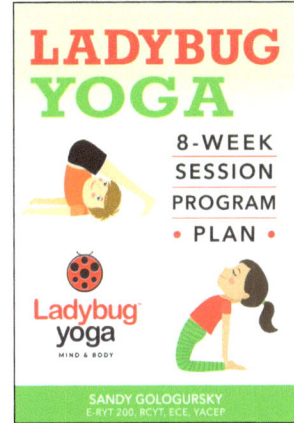

STEP-BY-STEP STARTUP GUIDE TO A CHILDREN'S YOGA BUSINESS

This is a very exciting time, as you are getting ready to embark on—and flourish in—your new venture! Your mind is exploding with amazing ideas, but you need assistance with the practical steps to take to get your business up and running—and have fun at the same time.

Let the **Step-by-Step Startup Guide to a Children's Yoga Business** show you how easy it can be to start your own thriving yoga business!

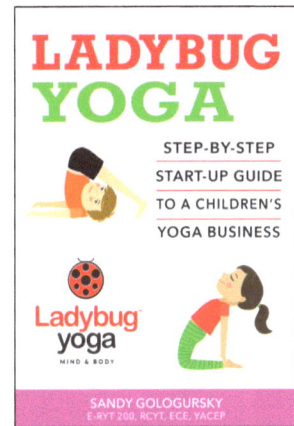

---

*Ladybug Yoga Children's Teacher Training is recognized as a Yoga Alliance Continuing Education Provider (YACEP). Registered Yoga Instructors can use this certification towards their Yoga Alliance Continuing Education (CE) hours. For more information on Ladybug Yoga certification, please contact Ladybug Yoga at contact@LadybugYoga.com or visit www.theLadybugYoga.com.